Ten Spices For Health And Longevity

By Valerie B. Lull, MH

Revised Edition

Library of Congress Control Number: 2016913990 CreateSpace Independent Publishing Platform, North Charleston, SC -- Valerie Lull

Ten Spices For Health And Longevity/ Valerie B. Lull, MH. —Revised Edition.

Contents

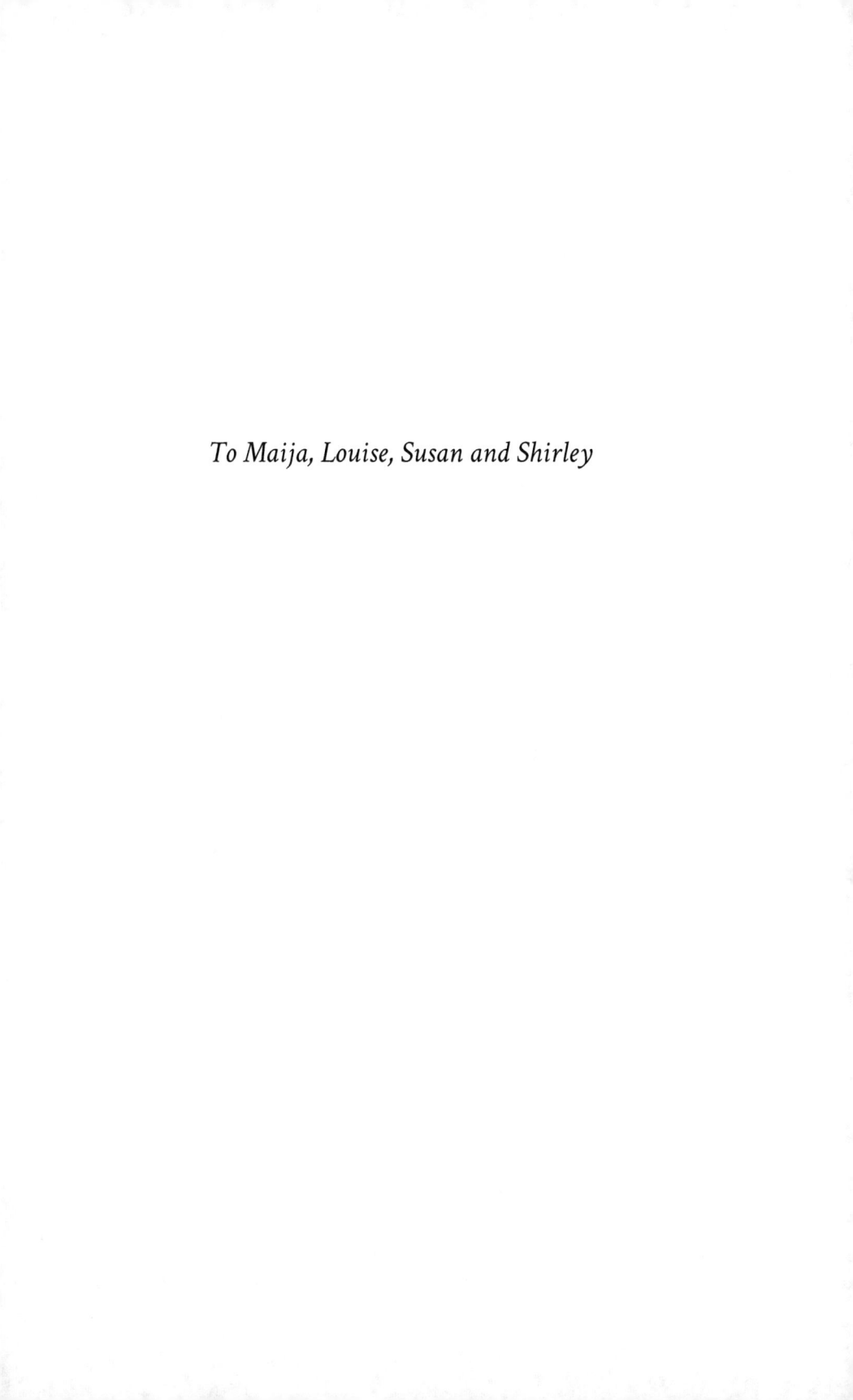

To Maija, Louise, Susan and Shirley

Why I Have Written this Book

I have always been interested in things that prevent disease and help people stay healthy. At the age of 58, I made a career change from mental health and studied to become a Master Herbalist. I learned many things that are simple and easy to do that help folks to stay healthy. I decided I wanted to share this information, especially with people that are interested in following a healthful lifestyle but don't know where to start.

My book is meant to be a guide to show how easy it is to do the simple things that can extend life and prevent disease. I started out with my first book, *Ten Healthy Teas,* and now I am delving into the world of healthful spices.

Many of the herbs and spices we are familiar with have culinary uses, as well as health properties, and are very inexpensive to buy. Many are as close as the produce department in the local market. Herbs and spices are used in everyday cooking, in teas, as supplements, and essential oils.

In writing this book I found it hard to narrow it down to 10 spices. There are so many good spices that have health benefits. There are many plants that are considered to be both herbs and spices; cinnamon for example. It is a popular spice used often in desserts and pastries, but it is also considered to be an herb that has medicinal uses. Most people put spices in the culinary category and don't think about their healing properties. They can be used to make teas and remedies that are therapeutic.

Healthy spices can also come in the form of essential oils. They are used extensively in aromatherapy, and massage therapy. Most essential oils cannot be taken orally. Be careful; some can be poisonous. Be sure you know what you are doing if you want to take essential oils orally. Always check with your health care provider before using essential oils, herbs or supplements.

You can improve your overall health by adding spices to your cooking, but sometimes that little extra is needed for a particular disorder.

I hope you will join me on this journey into the world of herbs and spices and vibrant health.

– Valerie Lull

CHAPTER 1

Cinnamon

Cinnamon is one spice that I really like. It can be used as an accent to a nutritious food, such as applesauce, or your morning oatmeal. It can be used alone in a tea. Cinnamon tastes good and it has health benefits.

There are two kinds of cinnamon, *cinnamomum cassia*, also called Chinese cinnamon, and *cinnamomum zeylanicum* known as Ceylon cinnamon. Cassia is from China and is the kind that is used the most in the United States. It is a sweeter and stronger tasting cinnamon than the Ceylon kind. However, research supports Ceylon cinnamon as having more health benefits [1].

Some people know Cinnamon as a winter spice. This is probably because it is used in so many of the foods prepared during the holiday season. Who can resist cinnamon buns, or baked apples with cinnamon, walnuts

---

[1] http://www.wsj.com/articles/SB10001424052702303376904579135502891970942

and raisins in them, or putting a cinnamon stick in a cup of hot tea or cocoa?

Cinnamon is one of a number of spices that are both an herb and a spice. It is good for both culinary and therapeutic purposes. There's some promising research on the use of cinnamon for controlling blood sugar. Recent findings seem to support the use of cinnamon for diabetes. It helps to bring down blood sugar [2] [3].

Cinnamon is also used for flatulence, muscle spasms, preventing vomiting, diarrhea, infections, colds, loss of appetite, impotence, lowering cholesterol and menopausal symptoms.

Some additional properties of cinnamon are that it is anti-inflammatory, anti-bacterial, ant repellent, and anti-fungal [4] [5].

But, don't go to the spice section in the supermarket and start downing bottles of cinnamon. You may get too much. The amount used in cooking is usually fine.

Cinnamon was used in ancient times. The Romans, who believed cinnamon was sacred, burned it at funerals. History tells us that Nero burned cinnamon at his wife's funeral. Cinnamon is also an important herb in the

---

[2] http://www.ncbi.nlm.nih.gov/pubmed/18552074

[3] http://www.ncbi.nlm.nih.gov/pubmed/24716174

[4] http://www.ncbi.nlm.nih.gov/pubmed/25629927

[5] http://www.ncbi.nlm.nih.gov/pubmed/27012624

Traditional Chinese Medicine compilation called *Materia Medica.*

In Chinese medicine, cinnamon was used to treat a wide variety of disorders characterized by intolerance to cold, cold limbs, weakness, soreness, coldness of the low back and knees, impotence, low libido, and loose bowel movements. Cinnamon is still used to treat digestive disorders that, according to traditional Chinese medical philosophy, are cold in nature. These may manifest as stomach pain and diarrhea. In the Chinese medical way of thinking the volatile oils in cinnamon have a mild stimulating action on digestion. They are thought to dispel gas, and relieve spasmodic pain in the stomach and intestines. There is no research in western medicine to verify this.

Also, in traditional Chinese medicine, the sliced twigs of the cinnamon tree can be used, and are in the category of warming diaphoretics; which is herbal language for an herb that makes you sweat. These twigs have been used for pain and stiffness in the muscles and joints with pain due to cold and damp. Cinnamon twigs can also be used as a guiding herb that leads other herbs to specific parts of the body.

There are other species of cinnamon, such as *C. Aburmuni.* These species are not used therapeutically because they are mild in nature. They are used primarily in cooking and baking.

Cinnamon can flavor fruits, vegetables, rice, and hot cocoa. Cinnamon sticks go well in both herbal tisanes and teas. Cinnamon suppresses the growth of E. coli and H. pylori. It may prevent or slow the progression of type II diabetes.

Cinnamon is often used as part of a tea blend to improve the taste of other less tasty herbs. It has powerful antibacterial properties that can be added to cold and flu remedies. Cinnamon can also make a tasty tea all by itself. Cinnamon is a good spice to keep on hand if the need for it arises.

Side Effects

Consuming large amounts of cinnamon over a long period of time may cause some people to bleed excessively. This is because the anti- platelet activity of the cinnamon. Cassia oil can irritate the skin.

Cinnamon can also cause an increase in heart rate, inflammation in the mouth, difficulty breathing, upset stomach, loose stools, and allergic reactions. Essential oil of cinnamon that is applied to the skin may cause burning and irritation. Women who are pregnant or nursing should avoid using cinnamon in medicinal doses.

Since the anti-platelet activity of cinnamon can thin the blood, it is not a good idea to take it before surgery or if you are taking blood thinning medications. Cinnamon may also interact with antibiotics. Always consult your health care practitioner.

Recipes

NOTE: Many spices and herbs can be used as teas. To make a tea, use 1 teaspoon of herb or spice, and 1 cup of boiling water. Leave it to steep for 2 to 10 minutes, depending on how strong you want it. Don't store the tea for more than 24 hours. An infusion is 1 oz. spice or herb and 1 pint of water that will steep for 20 minutes. A decoction is usually used for roots, bark and stems and is made in a saucepan. Enamel or stainless steel works best. Never use aluminum. It is made with 1 oz. bark, root or stems, and 1 pint of water. Simmer until ¼ of the water has evaporated. Strain the decoction and use. Do not store in the refrigerator for more than 24 hours.

Cinnamon Tea

Many fine teas are made with blends of cinnamon and other spices with fruits and herbs. Cinnamon alone can make a fine tea. It can also be added to teas that do not taste good to improve the flavor. Here is a simple recipe:

- Take 1 stick of cinnamon, use a small stick and break it in half per 1-2 cups of boiling water.

- Sweeten as desired. You can use honey, stevia or your own favorite sweetener. Agave syrup and maple syrup are other good options.

Add boiling water and steep for 10 minutes. Using powdered cinnamon will make the tea cloudy.

Breakfast Rice with Cinnamon

- 1 bowl of cooked rice: either white or brown is fine

- 1 teaspoon cinnamon

- 1 teaspoon brown sugar

- Butter: as much as desired and/or milk

Mix ingredients and enjoy. More cinnamon and brown sugar can be used if desired.

Additional Uses

Air freshener

Put a few drops of cinnamon essential oil on a cool light bulb so that it can diffuse throughout the room. Another way to freshen the air is to put some cinnamon in small dishes, and distribute them around your home. A third way to use cinnamon to freshen the air is to mix a few drops of cinnamon essential oil with water, put it in a spray bottle and spray it around the house. It helps to get rid of germs and unwanted odors.

Ant repellent

Sprinkle some cinnamon in places where the ants come in, as well as on their regular trails. You can also make a spray for this purpose. Put cinnamon essential oil and vinegar in a spray bottle. Use about 100 drops of cinnamon essential oil and add one cup of vinegar.

Incense

Cinnamon incense is available to burn in your home, or you can put some cinnamon in a dish that is heat proof and light it and burn it.

Massage

Mix a few drops of cinnamon essential oil with carrier oil, such as safflower oil or coconut oil, and use it for massage. It is warming to the body.

Moth repellent

Mix some broken cinnamon sticks with cloves and black peppercorns. Put them in little cloth sacks and hang them in your closet or any other place where you want to get rid of moths.

CHAPTER 2

Ginger

The spice known as ginger comes from the underground rhizome of the ginger plant, known botanically as *Zingiber officinale.* Ginger is another one of my favorite spices. I like to drink ginger tea on cool fall and winter mornings. It warms me up and helps my arthritis.

Ginger is used extensively in cakes, cookies and Asian cuisine. Besides gingers culinary uses, ginger is also useful for healing purposes. It was a favorite spice for cooking and healing in ancient China and Rome. In Chinese medicine it is considered a warming herb.

In both Traditional Chinese medicine and in Ayurveda (the medicine of India), ginger is mentioned in the earliest writings. It is used extensively in Traditional Chinese medicine for colds and for its usefulness in detoxifying the body and raising body heat.

In Chinese medicine ginger is called Gan-jiang for dried ginger and Sheg-jiang for fresh ginger. Juice squeezed from the root is used for burns and ginger is used in at least half of all Chinese medications. It is believed that ginger, used in moderation, can strengthen the lungs and kidneys.

You are traveling and have problems with motion sickness, ginger is a good remedy to have on hand [6] [7].

In addition to helping digestive problems ginger is anti-inflammatory. Ginger is good for upset stomach, nausea, body aches, arthritis, and motion sickness. Some folks find it relaxing and calming. Ginger is also used for morning sickness during pregnancy, though some doctors caution against using it. The caution against using ginger in pregnancy has not been clinically proven. Always check with your health care provider before taking ginger, especially if you are pregnant.

In the world of herbs, ginger has been used in herbal formulas to disguise the taste of other herbs that don't taste good. In some formulas it increases potency, which means it helps to speed up the action of the formula.

Ginger is thought to increase blood flow, helping to relieve abdominal cramps and bring on menstruation. Ginger has been used for the relief of pain from arthritis, coughs, bronchitis, chest pain, low back pain and stomach pain.

Ginger oil is used in massage blends. It has a spicy-woody odor. It warms the body and relaxes tight, sore

---

[6] http://www.ncbi.nlm.nih.gov/pubmed/23638927

[7] http://www.ncbi.nlm.nih.gov/pubmed/25789209

muscles. It is also useful for controlling nausea from chemotherapy. It improves digestion and can prevent indigestion.

Ginger combines well in herbal formulas and especially with turmeric, another anti-inflammatory and pain-relieving herb. Ginger is a carminative. That means it helps flatulence or intestinal gas. It is soothing and causes the intestinal tract to relax.

According to modern research, ginger possesses antioxidants and is anti-inflammatory. The anti-inflammatory effects of ginger are substances called gingerols. The gingerols help relieve pain from arthritis; both osteoarthritis and rheumatoid arthritis. Gingerols may inhibit the growth of colon cancer cells. Recent research also suggests that gingerols may also kill ovarian cancer cells. Ginger may also have anti-tumor properties.

Ginger may cause sweating, which is a good thing when folks have colds or the flu. Sweating aids in detoxifyingof the body. Fresh ginger seems to be more potent then dried ginger.

Side Effects

Do not take ginger if you are on a blood-thinning medication, or an aspirin regimen. People with heart problems, gallstones and diabetes should ask their doctors before starting to use ginger. In high doses ginger may cause heartburn, diarrhea and irritation of the mouth. Some of this may be avoided if the ginger is taken with meals.

Ginger may interact with some medications like warfarin (Coumadin), or clopidogrel (Plavix). In people with diabetes it may also lower blood sugar. Ginger may interact with blood pressure medications. Be sure to consult your doctor before using ginger for medicinal purposes and especially if you are pregnant.

Do not give ginger to children under two. If you want to give it to older children, consult your pediatrician for the right dosage.

Recipes

NOTE: Ginger can be used to improve the flavor of teas that do not taste good.

Ginger Ale Punch

- 1 Quart ginger ale
- 1 Quart apple or cranberry juice or cranberry apple juice
- A pinch of cinnamon

Mix ingredients. Chill and/or add ice. Serve and enjoy!

Fresh Ginger Tea

- 4-6 thin slices raw ginger, more for a stronger tea
- 1 1/2 - 2 cups water

- Juice from ½ a lemon

- 1-2 Tablespoon honey or sweetener of choice

Peel the ginger and slice thinly.

Boil the ginger in water for at least 10 minutes. For a stronger tea, allow it to boil for 20 minutes or more, and use more slices of ginger.

Remove from heat and add lemon and honey or sweetener of choice. Enjoy!

Ginger and Honey (for digestion)

- One piece of fresh ginger 3-4 inches' long

- 1 teaspoon of honey

- Water

Peel ginger. Put it in a blender with water to crush it. Remove from the blender and squeeze out the juice. Filter the juice. Add honey. Mix well and drink.

This recipe is good for food poisoning as well as for an upset stomach.

Additional Uses

Anti-inflammatory

Ginger extract has anti-inflammatory properties.

Bath

If you have sore muscles, arthritis, or fibromyalgia, you can take a soothing and detoxifying bath with rosemary and ginger combined.

Circulation

Ginger added to food aids the blood circulation.

Lemonade

Add ginger to your lemonade for an additional zing.

Lung congestion

A ginger poultice is good for lung congestion

Massage

Ginger can be blended with other oils to relieve sore muscles and cause relaxation.

CHAPTER 3

Cayenne

Cayenne, known in Latin as Capsicum annuum, is a member of the capsicium family. Cayenne is an interesting spice. It is part of the family of peppers, like jalapeno, habanero, chili peppers, bell peppers and more. It is known for its spicy heat and it will make you sweat. This makes it a good herb for removing toxins from your body.

Peppers are native to South and Central America. These cultures are famous for their spicy hot food. The early explorers introduced hot peppers to the rest of the world. The peoples of Europe, Africa and Asia used them to develop their own spicy dishes. They also developed medicinal uses as well as culinary uses for this herb.

Cayenne is hot, spicy and used a lot in cooking. The heat is caused by a substance called capsaicin. Capsaicin has been studied for its pain relieving properties, and cardiovascular benefits. Cayenne is also very effective for opening up congested nasal cavities.

Cayenne has vitamin A in it, along with beta-carotene. Some authorities feel it is helpful for asthma, osteoarthritis and rheumatoid arthritis. It is also an antioxidant that helps prevent free radicals that can lead to atherosclerosis, colon cancer, and diabetic problems like nerve damage and heart disease. Cayenne is rich in Vitamin C, and contains the minerals iron, copper and potassium.

Cayenne is used to fight pain. It inhibits a substance in the body called substance P, a substance that stimulates nerve fibers and causes pain [8].

Cayenne is being studied for the treatment of pain associated with psoriasis, arthritis, and diabetic neuropathy. Cayenne is useful for arthritis. There are many cream and ointment formulations on the market with capsaicin as the main ingredient that can be put on the areas that are painful.

Cayenne has some benefits for the cardiovascular system. They include lowering cholesterol, triglycerides, platelet aggregation and fibrin. Cultures where hot peppers like cayenne are used extensively have a lower rate of heart attack, stroke, and pulmonary embolism.

Cayenne can be good for heart health. Capsaicin, the active ingredient in cayenne, stimulates blood flow if it is taken on a regular basis [9].

---

[8] http://umm.edu/health/medical/altmed/herb/cayenne

[9] http://americannutritionassociation.org/newsletter/cayenne

The capsaicin in peppers is wonderful for clearing out the sinuses and very useful for coughs and colds. A tea made of hot cayenne pepper and garlic helps the sinuses drain and relieves congestion.

Cayenne has been used for losing weight. The heat generated by the consumption of the pepper produces the burning of calories. This is because thermogenesis is created, and oxygen consumption is increased for up to 20 minutes or more, after it is taken. One study showed that cayenne can suppress the appetite in folks that do not regularly eat spicy foods. It also showed that as a person gets used to the spice they become desensitized and the effect decreases [10].

Side Effects

Cayenne is in the nightshade family, and if you have problems consuming nightshades then it is better to stay away from cayenne.

Be careful using cayenne topically unless it is in a lotion, cream or ointment. It can cause burning and itching of the skin. Don't use on the sensitive skin around the eyes.

Very little research has been done regarding oral use of cayenne for children. It is probably best not to give it to them. Consult your health care provider.

[10] http://www.purdue.edu/newsroom/research/2011/110425MattesPepper.html

Stop cayenne 2 weeks before surgery. It may cause excessive bleeding. Always consult your health care practitioner.

Recipes

Cayenne Tea

- ½ to 1 teaspoon of cayenne pepper (depending on how strong you want it).
- 1 cup water
- Heat water to boiling. Pour it over some cayenne pepper in a cup.

Drink slowly and let it slide down your throat.

Garlic Broth with Chicken and Cayenne

(This is really good for clearing out your nasal passages if you have a cold or the flu.)

- 1 teaspoon cayenne pepper
- 1-2 teaspoon minced garlic
- 1-2 teaspoon chicken bullion

Add these three ingredients to 11/2 cups of boiling water. Stir and enjoy.

Cayenne and Green Bean Stir Fry

- 1 cup fresh sliced tomatoes
- ½ teaspoon cayenne pepper (more if desired)

- 2 cups green beans, fresh or frozen.

Toss together in a wok or frying pan. Cook 7-10 minutes depending on how crunchy you like your beans.

Serve and enjoy!

Cayenne Weight Loss Drink

- Cayenne pepper
- Lemon juice
- Sweetener of choice (stevia, agave, maple syrup, honey)

Mix in proportions as desired. Drink for weight loss.

Measure the ingredients into a large cup or a soup bowl with a handle on it. Pour boiling water over it and mix it up. Drink at your leisure.

Additional Uses

Discourage animals

Cayenne pepper can be useful to repel wildlife like squirrels, rabbits and deer.

Tea

Cayenne added to chicken soup will help clean out your sinuses. Cayenne can be made into a tea with horseradish for the same purpose.

CHAPTER 4

Sage

Now let's move from South America to the Mediterranean. There are many herbs that come from this part of the world, such as lavender, rosemary, sweet basil and thyme. They all belong to the *Lamiaceae* family. The Latin name for sage is *Salvia Officinalis* which means, "To save."

During the time of the bubonic plague in Europe, thieves developed a concoction containing sage that was called Four Thieves Vinegar, which was said to prevent them from getting the plague.

Sage was also used as a meat preservative before the days of refrigeration. The people in the Middle Ages thought that sage warded off evil spirits and the Emperor Charlemagne recommended it for cultivation. During the middle ages it was cultivated in monastery gardens and used for healing purposes.

According to folklore, sage is good for many things; nervous disorders, memory, digestive problems, mental disorders, Alzheimer's disease, and depression. In modern times research has been done regarding the use of sage for Alzheimer's and preliminary findings are promising [11].

Sage is anti-inflammatory and may help Type 2 diabetes. It has also been widely used for relieving the hot flashes of menopause. Sage has the properties of tonic, astringent, diaphoretic, and stimulant.

Sage oil is good for stiff muscles, rheumatism and neuralgia. Sage is sometimes used topically for eczema and skin injuries. Sage is also anti-viral, anti-fungal, and antibacterial. Sage is used in aromatherapy to relieve headaches, stress, nervousness and anxiety. Sage can soothe indigestion and it can be made into an herbal tea that can serve as a good mouthwash. Rubbing sage leaves on your teeth can whiten them and combat bad breath. It is good for gum disease and throat infections.

Sage has been used as a hot decoction for colds and flu, and it can act as a diaphoretic. This is good because the sweating helps your body to get rid of toxins. Sage has also been used as a cold infusion that can decrease sweating and it also can stop diarrhea.

Sage can dry up breast milk, so it is not recommended for a mother who is nursing, however it can be useful for a mother who is weaning an older baby. Sage is useful for treating the hot flashes that come with menopause.

---

[11] http://www.ncbi.nlm.nih.gov/pmc/articles/PMC4003706/

Sage comes in capsules, teas, oils, and tinctures. Sage tea can be blended with other herbs like lavender, mint, and catnip. Sage contains folic acid, pyridoxine, vitamin A, vitamin C, vitamin k, zinc, iron, calcium, copper, manganese, magnesium, potassium, and flavonoids. Sage has antioxidant properties that destroy free radicals.

Side Effects

The use of large quantities of sage can cause nervous irritation, convulsions, and death. It should not be used by people with epileptic conditions. It should not be used in pregnancy because it stimulates the uterus and may cause miscarriage. Sage can cause irritation and dry mouth.

Sage has a constituent called thujone and if sage is taken for a long period of time the thujone can cause confusion and an increase in heart rate. To avoid this, only take sage under a health care professional's guidance for a short period of time, like 1-2 weeks, then stop for a while. Be sure to talk to your health care provider about whether or not using sage is right for you. Sage can increase blood pressure in some people. It can interact with diabetic medicines, and sedative medicines. Proceed with caution and check it out with your health care provider.

Recipes

Sore Throat Gargle

- 1 tablespoon of dried sage leaves
- 1 pint boiling water

Bring to a boil and let it steep for about 15 minutes. Strain, and add honey or sweetener of choice. Use as a gargle twice a day.

Sage Tea

- 1 teaspoon dried sage
- 2 cups boiling water
- Lemon if desired

Add sage to the boiling water. Remove from the heat. Add honey, maple syrup or desired sweetener because sage alone tastes bitter.

> NOTE: Sage can be mixed with black tea for flavor and variety. Also, you can combine it with rosemary, thyme or lavender and some lemon zest. Experiment with different ingredients and see what you like best. An infusion is more concentrated than a tea. For an infusion add more sage and let it steep fora longer period of time. Infusions are usually used for medicinal purposes.

Sage and Fennel Tea

(good for sore throat, colds and flu)

- 1 ounce sage leaves
- ¾ ounces fennel seeds

- 1 cup water, boiled

Make a mixture of the sage leaves and fennel seeds. Use 1 ½ teaspoons of the mixture and pour the boiling water over it. Let it steep for 2-3 minutes. Drink it slowly and let it slide down your throat. A variation of this can be made using mint instead of fennel. Sweeteners and/or lemon can be added as desired

---

Additional Uses

After-shave

Sage has astringent properties and can be used as an after-shave.

Gargle

Sage tea can be mixed with a small amount of apple cider vinegar and used as a gargle for sore throats, laryngitis and tonsillitis.

Gray hair

In the past, sage was used to darken gray hair. It is good for your scalp and makes the hair feel soft and shiny.

Indigestion

Sage tea can be used for digestion problems and flatulence.

CHAPTER 5

Rosemary

Rosemary, *Rosmarinus officinalis*, is another herb from the Mediterranean area. It is in the mint family, *Lamiaceae*, and is an evergreen. Rosemary is used for flavoring food and beverages and is used in cosmetics. It is a useful herb for cooking meat, and is used often with lamb. Some recent research suggests that it has anti-cancer properties. Rosemary is anti-bacterial, anti-inflammatory, anti-fungal, and antiseptic.

Rosemary is known as the "herb of remembrance." The ancients used it for strengthening the memory. The first knowledge we have of rosemary dates back to around 5000 BCE. The Romans would put sprigs of rosemary on the graves of loved ones to show that they would be remembered. During the time of the Tudors in England, brides would wear rosemary to signify that they would not forget their families or the life they had before their marriage.

Pliny (23-79AD), Dioscorides, and Galen were famous healers in ancient times who wrote about rosemary. It was popular for flavoring meats during the

Middle Ages. Rosemary was thought to protect folks against the bubonic plague of the 1600's, and was mentioned in the writings of both Shakespeare and Sir Thomas Moore.

There is an old saying; "where rosemary flourishes the lady rules." However, husbands destroying the plant did not usually bring relief from their wives' rule. Rosemary was burned during religious ceremonies and in the rooms of the sick to purify the air.

Rosemary is historically credited with helping memory and recall. Ophelia in Shakespeare's Hamlet speaks of rosemary being for remembrance. Scholars in ancient Greece would wear wreaths of rosemary to help them in their exams.

In modern times, rosemary is recognized for its medicinal uses. It contains salicylic acid and is considered by many to be useful for arthritis. It is also used for skin problems, like dandruff. Rosemary is being researched for potential anti-cancer properties and may be useful for preventing and treating Alzheimer's disease.

Rosemary is popular to stimulate the hair follicles and help prevent premature balding, but there is no research to back it up. However, research does show that it is good for dandruff. Rosemary is used in folklore to reverse graying hair. The theory goes that it stimulates the roots of the hair and increases blood flow to the head. This promotes growth and prevents breakage.

Rosemary tea is useful for headaches, colds and depression. It is a tonic, astringent, diaphoretic, and is a stimulant. The oil can be used externally for gout and rheumatism. It is good for anxiety and it is good for mild memory impairment [12] [13].

Some of the nutritional benefits of rosemary include dietary fiber, Vitamins A, B-6, C, D, E and K, as well as pyridoxine, folic acid, pantothenic acid, and minerals like potassium, calcium, iron, manganese, copper and magnesium are also present but in minute amounts. It is high in antioxidants. Rosemary contains a substance called rosmarinic acid, which is anti-inflammatory. Rosemary also contains fiber.

Rosemary contains substances that stimulate the immune system and help digestion. It can reduce the severity of asthma attacks, and it appears to increase blood flow to the brain, improving concentration. Another interesting property of rosemary is that it seems to make hair grow faster for rats. Whether or not this extends to humans is not proven.

Rosemary is considered good for staving off the aging process because it is used as an ingredient in skin preparations and is known to rejuvenate the skin [14].

---

[12] http://www.ncbi.nlm.nih.gov/pubmed/27133263

[13] http://www.ncbi.nlm.nih.gov/pubmed/27113201

[14] http://www.ncbi.nlm.nih.gov/pubmed/27210890

It sharpens mental clarity and stimulates the function of the brain. For many people rosemary is good for long-term memory. It has also been used by students to help them retain the memory of their studies for longer periods of time.

Rosemary cleanses the system by helping the liver to function better. Rosemary can calm an upset stomach and relieve muscle pain. It can help you fight stress and anxiety by helping you to relax. It can be applied topically for arthritis, sore muscles, and pain in the joints and muscles. It is good for indigestion, and helps prevent food borne illness if it is taken with meat or eggs. It is also a mild diuretic and assists kidney function.

Side Effects

The use of rosemary as a medicine for children does not have any research to back it up. Do not give it to children under 18 years of age. It is safe for children to eat foods that have rosemary spice in them.

Do not take more than 6g of dried rosemary per day. Do not take rosemary oil orally because it is toxic. Caution is recommended for pregnant women, because rosemary can cause miscarriage. It is also not recommended for nursing mothers.

Do not take rosemary if you have high blood pressure, ulcerative colitis, or Crohn's disease. Rosemary may interfere with blood thinners like Warfarin, ACE inhibitors for high blood pressure, and diabetes medicines. As always, check with your health care provider before using rosemary therapeutically.

Recipes

Rosemary Tea

- 1 teaspoon rosemary

- 1 cup boiling water

Steep for 4-5 minutes, or longer if you want it stronger. Drink and enjoy.

> NOTE: you can combine the rosemary with lavender or thyme to make a tasty beverage. You can also add lemon and/or honey.

Biscuits with Rosemary

- 2 cup baking mix (biscuit mix is good)

- ½ teaspoon sugar

- ¾ cup milk

- 2 tablespoons Butter

- 2 teaspoon dried rosemary, crumbled up

Mix ingredients with baking mix. Add more or less milk as need to get soft dough. Roll out dough to ½ inch thickness, on a lightly floured surface. Cut it into biscuit rounds and put them on a greased and floured baking sheet. Bake according to directions on the baking mix package.

Potatoes with Rosemary

- 1 pound potatoes (Yukon Gold is good but you can use any kind).

- 2 tablespoons olive oil

- 1 teaspoon salt

- 5 teaspoons chopped fresh rosemary with stems removed (you can use dried rosemary but there is nothing like the taste of fresh)

- ½ t ground pepper (more or less as desired)

Chop the potatoes into small cubes and completely coat them with the olive oil. Add rosemary, salt and pepper. Garlic may be added if desired. Stir well. Turn into a baking dish that has been sprayed with a non-stick spray. Use a fairly large dish so potatoes are spread out instead of bunched on top of each other, (unless you want to stir them more often while they are baking). Bake for 45 minutes, stirring them once or twice until golden brown. Use the broiler towards the end if you like them crispy. Remove from the oven and serve. This goes well with steak.

Additional Uses

Air freshener

Rosemary can be used as an air freshener. You can make potpourri with rosemary.

Baldness

According to folklore, rosemary is a remedy for baldness, though there is no scientific evidence for this.

Bath

For a soothing bath for sore muscles you can take 2 cups of rosemary and make an infusion. Let it steep for 20 minutes and add to your bath. Epsom salts can also be added if desired.

Congestion

For congestion in the respiratory tract, breathe in the scent of rosemary oil. You can also boil rosemary in water, place it in a bowl, put a towel over your head and breathe in the steam. This is good for stuffed up sinuses.

Dandruff

A strong infusion of nettle leaf and rosemary can be used as an herbal rinse for hair that fights dandruff. It can speed hair growth and condition your scalp. Use it as a rinse after washing.

Diffuser

You can use rosemary essential oil in a diffuser. It is said to help folks maintain their focus, so good to use in the workplace.

Eyes

Use wet rosemary tea bags for puffy eyes. Apply bags to your eyelids for 10 minutes. Wash your face afterwards to prevent skin staining.

Mouthwash

Rosemary can be used as a mouthwash. Steep some rosemary in 2 c of water, strain and use. It may be refrigerated.

CHAPTER 6

Thyme

Thyme, *Thymus Vulgaris*, is another Mediterranean herb that is popular. It is a perennial plant that is used in Italian, Greek, Spanish and French cooking. There are several varieties of thyme. I like lemon thyme. Thyme has many medicinal uses such as treating infections and using thyme oil in cough syrups. It is antiseptic, antibacterial and antifungal.

Thyme is another spice that was used a lot by the Greeks and Romans. In Roman times thyme was used for the culture of bees. The Egyptians used it in embalming, to preserve the bodies of their pharaohs and other important people. They also used it in their baths. They used it for depression, and to lift their mood.

Thyme was considered by the Romans to be an antidote for poison. It was a favorite of the emperors for that reason, and a bath in warm water with thyme was thought to stop the effects of poison if it was accidentally consumed.

In the Middle Ages, thyme was grown in monastery gardens for use in cooking. Thyme was used to preserve meat before refrigeration and thyme oil was used to treat consumption. When the bubonic plague struck in the 14th century, people used thyme for relief and for prevention. The famous herbalist Culpeper suggested using thyme for nightmares. In a Victorian myth, it states that a patch of thyme was a place where fairies had danced during the night.

Thyme can help digestive problems[15] and prevent flatulence. It is antispasmodic and relieves menstrual cramping. Tea made of thyme can help a hangover, and it is often used for sore throats, colds, and reducing respiratory inflammation. It has also been used to clear congestion.

Thyme is useful for relieving bronchitis. It has been used as a base for formulating a mouthwash that is used in treating dental cavities and gingivitis. Thyme contains antioxidants, one of which is lutein. Lutein is good for your eyes. It also contains B-complex vitamins, vitamins A, K, E, and C and folic acid, as well as calcium, potassium. Thyme contains trace amounts of manganese, magnesium, iron, and selenium.

Thyme can be used for pink eye or conjunctivitis. It works to eliminate lice and can help with gastroenteritis. Thyme is good for fatigue, and stress. Thyme contains antioxidants and flavonoids that neutralize free radicals

---

[15] http://www.ncbi.nlm.nih.gov/pubmed/27175199

in the body. Thyme is useful for Alzheimer's disease, arthritis, and is an anti-fungal that is good for athlete's foot. Thyme tea is good for emphysema, asthma, and hay fever.

Thyme combats parasites such as hookworms and tapeworms. Thyme is good for reducing the pain of arthritis. Hot thyme tea can be used to induce menstruation. For this reason, it should not be used during pregnancy.

Thyme is a diaphoretic, which means it induces perspiration, and a febrifuge, which means it brings down a fever.

Thyme is a good herb and is useful for a lot of things, even hand sanitizer and acne treatment.

Side Effects

If you have Allergic Reactions to plants in the *Lamiaceae* family, avoid drinking tea made from thyme. Some of the side effects of large doses of thyme include heartburn, nausea, diarrhea, upset stomach, headache and dizziness.

Folks are cautioned to be careful about drinking thyme tea if they have a history of heart disease, peptic ulcers and gastrointestinal problems. The amounts used in cooking are considered to be safe.

There has not been a lot of research on the effects of thyme on pregnant women or nursing mothers. If you are pregnant consult your health care provider before using thyme tea or supplements.

Recipes

Thyme Tea Recipe

- 1 teaspoon of dried thyme leaves, or 2 teaspoons fresh thyme leaves
- 2 cups of boiled fresh water.

Let it steep for 4-5 minutes.

Sweeten to taste with honey, or stevia, or agave syrup.

For variation use lemon thyme, or add lemon to regular thyme.

Rice with Lemon Thyme

- 1 tablespoon butter
- 1 cup rice, brown or white is ok. I prefer brown.
- 1 can of organic, chicken broth
- 1 tablespoon lemon juice
- 1 tablespoon Thyme, fresh is preferred

Melt the butter and stir in the rice. Cook rice, until browned, for about 5 minutes. Mix the chicken broth, lemon juice and thyme into the rice. Cover and reduce heat to low. Cook until all the liquid has been absorbed. Fluff and serve. For variations add chopped onion, or olives, or shredded chicken, or parmesan cheese.

Rice with Chicken and Thyme

- 2 cups cooked rice (I use brown rice, but you can use white)
- 1 or 2 cups of fresh mushrooms (depending on how much you like mushrooms)
- 3 teaspoons olive oil
- 1 onion diced
- 2 teaspoons ground thyme
- ½ teaspoon poultry seasoning
- Salt and pepper to taste
- 1 ½ cups diced chicken cooked
- ½ cup chicken stock
- ½ cup sour cream
- ½ cup grated parmesan
- 2cups cheese (A Mexican blend is good, also cheddar works)

Cook the rice and preheat the oven to 375 degrees.

Slice the mushrooms and put them in a pan with 2 teaspoons of the olive oil and sauté. Add mushrooms and continue to sauté. Add thyme, poultry seasoning, salt, and pepper. Let the flavors mix and cook for a minute or so. Dice the chicken. In a bowl, add the sauté mix and chicken. Add the rice. Mix. In a separate bowl, mix together the sour cream, chicken stock, parmesan cheese and 1 cup of the grated cheese. Stir it into the mushroom and rice mixture. Use the remaining olive oil to grease a 2-quart casserole dish. Put the mixture into the casserole dish. Bake for 25 minutes. Sprinkle the rest of the cheese on top of the casserole and bake until the cheese starts to brown. Remove from the oven and serve hot.

Additional Uses

Antiseptic

Fresh thyme leaves can be crushed and applied to cuts and wounds. Thyme is a natural antiseptic.

Bath

Thyme can be added to a hot bath to relieve the pain of body aches.

Colds and bronchitis

Thyme can be added to hot water when it is steaming. Inhaling the steam can help folks suffering from colds and bronchitis. It clears the respiratory airways.

Cosmetic

Thyme has a lot of hygienic and cosmetic uses. It is added to shampoos, and soaps.

Cuts and wounds

Strong thyme tea can be used as an antiseptic on external cuts and wounds.

Digestion remedy

Mix equal amounts of thyme, red clover, sage and rosemary. If you have nausea, add some sliced ginger.

Fungus

A tea made from thyme can be externally applied with a cotton ball to athlete's foot and toenail fungus.

Gum disease

Thyme tea is a good gargle or rinse for gum disease.

Infected eyes

Thyme tea bags can be used like a compress on infected eyes.

CHAPTER 7

Basil

Basil *Ocimum basilicum* is also known as sweet basil. This is different from holy basil, *Basilicum sanctum*, which is used extensively in India and is a related species. Basil and its variations are thought to have originated in India. Basil is used extensively in Ayurvedic medicine, the ancient medicine of India. It was also used in Chinese medicine to promote blood circulation after birth, heal kidney problems and relieve stomach cramps. A variety of basil called Holy Basil is considered sacred in India.

In Greek lore, basil represents hatred and in European lore it is sometimes called the symbol of Satan. The famous herbalist Culpeper cites "Hilarios," a French physician, as saying that basil breeds scorpions in the brain. Basil is placed in the hands of the dead in Europe and in India it is placed in the mouth of the dying to make sure they reach God. The ancient Egyptians thought it would open the gates of heaven for a person who had died.

Basil has been used to help bronchitis, osteoarthritis, anxiety, insomnia, stress, indigestion and general pain. Basil helps lower blood pressure, ease tension and stress, relieve spasms, act as a detoxification agent, and as a cleanser for the blood. It is said to lower blood sugar. Basil may ease anxiety, work as an anti-inflammatory, lower cholesterol, and act as an adaptive, which means it can help the body adapt and bounce back.

According to folk lore the benefits of basil include: stimulating the brain, clearing the mind, aiding concentration, increasing endurance and stamina, resisting infection, improving blood circulation, and increasing the production of breast milk. Basil has a mild soothing effect that helps with nervousness and irritability, anxiety, depression and insomnia.

Basil can ease constipation, stomach cramps, indigestion, vomiting, and nausea from chemotherapy. It can help whooping cough, hiccups, headaches and migraines, depression, fevers, colds, influenza, coughs and sinusitis. It can ease cramps in the uterus and intestines, aid insomnia and it has also been used to treat epilepsy; though I wouldn't recommend it for epilepsy without consulting a physician first.

Basil is good for gastrointestinal problems, like flatulence, cramping, colic, nausea and vomiting, worms, and parasites. Basil can be used for migraines, whooping cough, skin disorders, and as an insect repellent, as well as for insect bites. Basil is sometimes used for arthritis and rheumatism. It is antibacterial, and antiseptic.

There are a number of cultures where basil is used to promote menstruation, and induce labor. Some think it is an aphrodisiac; however, there is no scientific evidence for this. Basil is anti-inflammatory and brings relief to things like aches and pains and inflamed bowels.

Basil contains a lot of nutrients. Among them are Vitamins A, C, K, iron, calcium, fiber, manganese, copper, magnesium, flavonoids and volatile oils. Basil essential oil will slow the growth of bad bacteria like staphylococcus that have become resistant to antibiotics. It also contains protein, and fiber.

Basil is a carminative, which means it is good for flatulence, and it is also good for fevers, and for catarrh. It helps genito-urinary disorders and helps to relieve constipation. Basil oil works against mosquitoes and flies. It has been used as an antidote for poison, for French liquors, perfumes, and as a gourmet seasoning.

Side Effects

Sweet basil has been known to enhance the effect of insulin and medicines that lower blood glucose. People with diabetes should be cautious with basil and consult with their health care provider.

Pregnant and nursing women should not use basil in larger amounts than that found in food. Always consult your health care practitioner.

Recipes

Basil Tea

- 1 cup boiling water

- 1 teaspoon dried basil or 2 teaspoons fresh

Pour boiling water over basil leaves and steep for 5 minutes. You can steep for a longer or shorter period of time depending on how strong you want it. For variation you can add lemon or lemon peel as desired. Strain, drink and enjoy.

For an infusion, steep it for 15 minutes. Do not have more than 2 cups of the infusion a day and do not take it for more than ten days without a break for several days.

Tomato Rice Basil soup

- 1 can diced tomatoes

- 2/3 cups cooked rice (I prefer brown but white is ok)

- 4 cups tomato juice

- 12 leaves of fresh basil

- 1 cup whipping cream

- ½ cup olive oil (or butter if you prefer)

- Salt and pepper to taste

Puree the tomatoes, basil and tomato juice and simmer for 30 minutes. Stir in a lot of cream, butter or olive oil. Season as desired. Let soup simmer for 5-10 minutes and serve.

Additional Uses

Asthma and bronchitis

The essential oil of basil can be used as a chest rub.

Bath

Five or ten drops of basil essential oil can be added to bath water for relaxation.

Cold and bronchitis

The decoction of basil mixed with honey and ginger is an effective remedy for asthma, influenza, cough, cold and bronchitis

Foot bath

Pour boiling water over basil leaves for a pain-relieving foot-bath.

Headache

Rub crushed basil leaves into your temples to relieve headaches.

Insect bites

Fresh, crushed leaves can be used for insect bites by rubbing the leaves on the bites to reduce inflammation and itching.

Insect repellent

The essential oil of basil can be applied externally as an insect repellent.

Inhalation

For head colds, the steam from basil leaves that have been in boiling water can be inhaled.

Warts

Basil leaves have traditionally been used to remove warts.

CHAPTER 8

Oregano

Yet another herb from the Mediterranean area of the world, oregano, is known as *Oreganum vulgare* in Latin. It also comes from the Lamiaceae family, which is also known as the mint family. The mint family is a large family of plants that includes sage, rosemary, thyme, marjoram and lemon balm.

The Greeks believed Aphrodite invented oregano to make man's life happier. They also put it on graves to give the departed spirits peace. Hippocrates used Oregano for stomach and respiratory disorders. The Romans adopted it from the Greeks and it spread to Europe and North Africa. It was used to spice meat and fish and it was used as a flavoring for wine.

Oregano was used in China as a medicinal herb for fever, vomiting, diarrhea, and itchy skin. In the United States, oregano was not common until after WW II when the soldiers came back from the war. It was mostly associated with pizza.

Oregano is antibacterial, antibiotic, antiviral and antifungal. The oregano oil is an especially strong antibacterial, and it is an antioxidant. It contains Vitamins C, E, and K as well as magnesium, calcium, several of the B vitamins, iron, potassium, and Vitamin A.

Oregano stimulates bile flow and relieves flatulence. It is antiseptic and often used for coughs, tonsillitis, bronchitis and asthma. It is used by herbalists for women's issues and can be applied topically to a toothache and aching joints.

Oregano has been used as a disinfectant and to relieve itchy skin. Oregano oil is very potent and is also anti-microbial. It helps kill intestinal parasites. It has been used for fungal infections like Candida. It has also been used for diarrhea, nausea, jaundice, and vomiting.

Oregano can be used to get rid of head lice. Oregano is an antioxidant that helps to slow down age related problems like, degeneration of the muscles. According to researchers, a tablespoon of fresh oregano contains as many antioxidants as a medium sized apple. Oregano is used for aging related diseases such as heart disease, high blood pressure, macular degeneration and geriatric muscle deterioration.

Oregano has been used for colds, as a decongestant, for a sore throat, and for infected sinuses. It acts as an anti-inflammatory and can be used for coughs. Oregano is often used for digestive complaints, such as an upset stomach, and diarrhea. It can kill parasites. Oregano is good for relieving minor aches and pains. It is useful for skin problems like fungal infections and nail fungus. Oregano oil is used for menstrual problems in women. Oregano is known for strengthening the immune system.

Oregano has culinary uses and is used in Italian dishes for seasoning. It is a standard spice for pizza.

Side Effects

Do not use on sensitive or broken skin. If Oregano is taken in doses that are too high, it can cause hives and itching.

Oregano for medicinal purposes is not recommended for pregnant or nursing women, or for children. Always seek guidance from your health care practitioner.

If oil of oregano is used for a long time it may interfere with the absorption of iron by the body. Take the dosage recommended by your health care provider.

Be careful using oregano for children. Start with small doses. Be sure to discuss it with your pediatrician before starting use.

Recipes

Oregano Tea

- 1 ½ teaspoons dried oregano leaves, or 2 ½ teaspoons fresh leaves

- 8 ounces boiling water
- 1 teaspoon honey (or sweetener of choice).

Place oregano leaves in boiling water and steep for 5 minutes. Steeping it longer will cause the tea to be bitter.

Strain into a mug. Add sweetener to taste. Stir and drink.

Oregano tea is good for sore throats and colds.

Variation for sinus congestion; skip the honey and add a drop or two of lime juice.

Meatball Soup with Fresh Oregano

- 5 cups vegetable broth
- 2 carrots diced
- 2 stalks celery diced
- 1 ½ teaspoons cumin
- 2 tablespoons chopped oregano
- ¼ teaspoon salt
- ¼ teaspoon pepper

Turkey Meatballs (you can get prepared meatballs at the market or you can make your own)

Heat broth, carrots and celery in a covered pot until it comes to a boil. Add the meatballs to the soup. Reduce heat to a simmer and cook until the carrots are tender. Stir in the fresh oregano. Oregano is best fresh, although dried can be used. For a variation add a half cup of brown rice, if desired.

Additional Uses

Add to meat

Adding oregano to meat before cooking can reduce toxic compounds.

Athlete's foot

Massage oregano oil into the feet. Add a drop or two to your socks and shoes.

Gargle

Oregano is used as a gargle for a sore tooth or a sore throat.

Hand wash

Add a few drops to liquid soap for washing your hands to fight germs and bacteria on your hands.

Head Lice

Add a couple of drops of oregano oil to shampoo to wash your head and scalp.

Mouthwash

A useful mouthwash can be made by adding a few drops to water and swishing through the mouth. It will destroy bad bacteria that grow in the mouth and help prevent tooth decay.

Sinus infection

For a sinus infection, inhale the steam from a bowl of hot water with a few drops of oregano oil in it.

Sinusitis

For sinusitis or sore throats, you can put 2-3 drops under your tongue using a medicine dropper.

Sore throat

For a sore throat put 2-3 drops of oregano oil in orange juice.

CHAPTER 9

Turmeric

The Latin name for turmeric is *Curcuma Longa*. It is a member of the ginger family *Zingiberaceae*. It comes from Asia and is used extensively in India. It has a bright yellow color and is used for curries, rice, and chutneys. It is also used as a dye for cloth. Turmeric gives mustard its yellow color and has many medicinal uses. It is sometimes called Indian saffron because its deep yellow color is similar to that of saffron.

Turmeric originated in Indonesia and Southern India and has been used for thousands of years. It was a highly regarded herb in Ayurvedic medicine. Arab traders brought it to Europe in the 13th century. In Traditional Chinese medicine it was used for depression. In the western world it was not popular until modern times when studies showed it was helpful for memory problems as well as a number of other conditions.

Scientists think that Turmeric is useful for Alzheimer's disease [16].

In India there is a very low incidence of this disease. In studies with mice turmeric appears to slow progression of this disease by slowing or preventing the formation of the Amyloid-B plaques in the brain that are characteristic of Alzheimer's disease [17].

Curcumin is the main constituent of turmeric which gives it the yellow color and it contains anti-inflammatory, antiseptic, antibacterial, and antioxidant properties. Turmeric has the potential to help colitis, and neutralize toxins in smoke.

Turmeric is very good for detoxifying the liver. Turmeric is a natural pain killer and it can help psoriasis and other skin diseases. Turmeric can be used for heartburn, diarrhea, stomach bloating, headaches, bronchitis, colds, lung infections, fibromyalgia, leprosy, fever and menstrual problems. It can be used for water retention, worms, kidney problems, flatulence.

Turmeric is very nutritious, containing vitamins C, E, and K as well as minerals such as sodium, calcium, copper potassium, iron, magnesium and zinc.

Curcumin is an antioxidant and that can neutralize free radicals that can cause damage in the body such as coronary artery disease, stroke and hypertension. It is a

---

[16] http://www.ncbi.nlm.nih.gov/pubmed/26420724

[17] http://www.ncbi.nlm.nih.gov/pubmed/26420724

useful herb that helps many chronic diseases like arthritis, heart disease, and stroke. Epidemiological studies suggest that the frequent use of turmeric can lower the incidence of breast, prostate, lung, and colon cancer. Turmeric supports the liver.

Side Effects

People who have gallstones or bile obstruction should not take turmeric. Also, pregnant women should consult their doctor before taking turmeric in medicinal doses. Turmeric may exacerbate problems with stomach ulcers. People should always consult their health care provider, especially if they have serious heart and liver problems.

Turmeric can cause nausea and diarrhea with long-term use. Turmeric may interfere with some medicines like aspirin, NSAID's, statins, diabetes drugs, blood pressure drugs and blood thinners. Don't give turmeric to children unless your pediatrician recommends it.

Recipes

Turmeric Tea

- 1 cup water
- 1 teaspoon turmeric
- lemon and/or honey to taste

Boil the water, add the turmeric and simmer for 10 minutes. Strain into a mug with a cheesecloth and add honey and/or lemon to taste.

This tea is good if you feel you are catching a cold or the flu. It also lessens inflammation.

Longevity Tea

- 1 teaspoon turmeric powder

- 4 cups water

Boil water and add turmeric. Let it simmer for 10 minutes, strain, and add ginger and/or honey to taste.

Turmeric Milk (good for relaxation)

- 1 cup coconut milk

- ½ teaspoon ground turmeric

- 2 teaspoons sweetener of choice (honey, agave, maple syrup, stevia)

- ½ cinnamon stick, or ground cinnamon

- Pinch black pepper

Put the turmeric and milk into a saucepan and bring it to a boil. Stir to combine. Reduce the heat and simmer 20-30 minutes. Strain if necessary. Add sweetener and cinnamon. Add a pinch of black pepper and/or vanilla if desired. Serves 1

Additional Uses

Cold or flu

Mix 1 teaspoon of turmeric powder in a glass of milk and drink.

Cuts and burns

Turmeric powder sprinkled on a cut or burn can speed up the healing process.

Curry powder

Blend your own secret recipe.

Dye Easter eggs

Turmeric is a dye and can be used for numerous things.

Face mask

Mix some turmeric with yogurt and honey. Apply to the skin for 20 minutes.

Homemade soap

Turmeric can add color to the soap and it is good for your skin.

Scrambled eggs or tofu

Add a pinch of turmeric to add to the flavor.

Sunburn

A paste made of turmeric can be applied to sunburn. It is also used in sunscreens.

CHAPTER 10

Clove

Clove, in the Latin classification is called *Syzugium aromaticum*. Clove is a member of the *Myrtacea* family. Clove trees originated in the Spice Islands and now cloves are grown all over the world.

The clove comes from the dried flower bud of the clove tree. Cloves are used extensively in cooking and are also used for medicinal remedies. The name clove came from the French word *clov*, which means nail. This is because a clove resembles a nail.

Archeologists have found cloves in a ceramic vessel in Syria, dating back to approximately the 3rd century BCE. In 200 B.C cloves came to China from Java. The emperor required that his visitors take a clove and hold it in their mouth to freshen their breath before an audience with him. The Romans used cloves for fragrance and perfume.

In the middle ages, Europeans used cloves to preserve and flavor food. In the 16th century Magellan sailed around the world and claimed the Spice Islands for

Portugal. In the 17th century the Dutch took over the clove business from the Portuguese and destroyed all clove trees except for those on two islands. They did it so that they could maintain their monopoly in the clove trade. In the second half of the 18th century the French smuggled cloves from the East Indies and took them to the new world, breaking the Dutch monopoly. Cloves are mentioned in the *Arabian Nights* where the Muslims traded with India for cloves.

Cloves used for medicinal purposes are perhaps best known for relieving the pain of a toothache if you are unable to get to a dentist right away. Cloves have been used for acne, and other skin conditions. Cloves are thought to relax the muscle lining of the stomach thereby bringing relief for digestive problems such as acid reflux.

Clove tea is used for bloating and gas as well as nausea and diarrhea. Cloves are used for toenail fungus and are good for inflammation of the mouth and throat. The oils, flower buds, leaves and stems are used to make medicine. Cloves are anti-fungal, antiseptic, antiviral, anesthetic, and are considered to be an aphrodisiac. Cloves are used for coughs, asthma and headaches.

Cloves are diaphoretic and can help relieve colds by causing perspiration for folks with fevers, sore throats and flu. In the past they were taken for whooping cough. Cloves are good for mouth ulcers and sore gums. A gargle can be used for a sore throat. Cloves can relieve nausea and vomiting as well as flatulence. Clove oil can be applied to the skin for cuts and scrapes.

Side Effects

Cloves are generally regarded as safe. Children should not take clove oil in excess as it can cause serious health problems such as seizures and liver damage. Clove oil is safe when applied to the skin and mouth sparingly. Inhaling the smoke from clove cigarettes is not safe and can cause breathing problems and lung infections.

Dried clove can cause irritation of the mouth, damage to the dental tissues and it is unsafe to inject clove oil into the veins. Pregnant and nursing women can take cloves in normal amounts in food but should not use it as a medicine. Always consult your physician before using cloves as a medicine.

Clove seems to slow the clotting of the blood so it should not be taken if you are on blood thinners, or for 2 weeks before surgery. Some people are allergic to cloves. Again, talk it over with your doctor. Be careful about giving small children a clove to suck on. It can be a choking hazard.

Recipes

Clove Tea

- 1 t crushed clove in a tea bag or infuser

- 1 C of boiling water

To prepare a clove tea, take a tea bag or infuser and fill it with crushed cloves. Let it steep, covered in a cup of water, for 8 to 10 minutes. Milk and sweetener can be added as desired. Cloves are often used in Chai teas.

Clove Tea for Respiratory Congestion

- 2 cloves
- 1 stick cinnamon
- Crushed cardamom seeds (1 or 2 seeds will do)
- 1 black tea bag
- 1 to 2 cups of water (depending on the size of your mug)

Place cloves, cinnamon and cardamom in an infuser. Place in a mug with boiling water and steep for 1 minute (steep longer for a stronger brew.)

Pumpkin Cookies with Clove, Cinnamon and Nutmeg

- 1 cup pumpkin
- ½ cup white sugar
- ½ cup brown sugar
- 1 egg
- 2 cup flour
- 2 teaspoons baking powder
- 2 teaspoons cinnamon
- ¼ teaspoon clove
- ¼ teaspoon nutmeg
- ½ teaspoon salt

- ½ teaspoon baking soda
- 1 teaspoon milk
- 1 teaspoon vanilla
- 2 cups semi-sweet chocolate chips
- ½ cup walnuts (if desired)

Combine pumpkin, sugar, oil and egg. Mix well. In a separate bowl add flour, baking powder, spices, salt, and baking soda. Combine the two mixtures. Add vanilla, chocolate chips and nuts. Drop on a greased cookie sheet and bake at 350 degrees for 10 to 12 minutes or until golden brown and firm.

Additional Uses

Acne

For acne, make a paste of clove powder and honey and apply to the affected area.

Bad Breath

Chewing on cloves can relieve bad breath.

Cough

Chewing a clove with salt can relieve coughing.

Earache

For an earache, mix clove oil and sesame oil. Warm the mixture and put 2-3 drops in the ear.

Indigestion

Drinking clove tea after a meal can ease indigestion.

Insect repellent

Clove oil diluted in a solution of water makes a good insect repellent.

Nausea

A cup of clove tea can relieve nausea and digestive problems.

Stomach ache

Clove oil taken with sugar is good for a stomach ache.

Throat congestion

Chewing a roasted clove is good for throat congestion. It is good for inflammation of the pharynx.

Toenail fungus

Apply clove oil directly to the skin or nails. The clove oil can be diluted with olive oil if you have sensitive skin.

Toothache

Press a clove between the jaws at the site of the toothache to ease pain.

Warts

Put a couple of drops of clove oil on a cotton ball or Band-Aid and place it over a wart. Change it every day. After 3-4 weeks the wart should disappear.

For Further Reading

- Aggarwal, Bharat, B., *Healing Spices How to use 50 Everyday Spices to Boost Health and Beat Disease*, 2011

- David, Elizabeth, *Spices, Salt and Aromatics in the English Kitchen*, Penguin Books, New York, 1976

- Dalby, Andrew, *Dangerous Tastes; the Story of Spices*, University of California Press, Berkeley, 2000

- Hemphill, Ian, *Spice and Herb Bible, 3rd edition*, Robert Rose Publisher, Toronto Ontario Canada, 2014

- Keay, John, *The Spice Route; A History*, University of California Press, Berkeley, 2006

- Little, Brenda, *The Complete Book of Herbs & Spices*, Silverleaf Press, Utah, 2006

- Simonds, Nina, *Spices of Life: Simple and delicious recipes for great health*, Alfred A. Knopf, New York, 2005

- Stanway, Penny, *The Miracle of Spices, Practical Tips for Health and Home,* Watkins Publishing, London, 2013

- Turner, Jack, *The History of a Temptation: Spice,* Vintage Books, New York, 2004

If you enjoyed this book write a review for Amazon and Goodreads.

Send me an e-mail with your comments and check out my website and blog.

- E-mail: *valerielull923@gmail.com*

- Check out my website, *www.valerielull.com*

- Check out my blog at *simplewaystostayhealthy.wordpress.com*

Other books by Valerie Lull are

- *Ten Healthy Teas*

- *The Sweet Side of the Stinking Rose: How to Use Garlic to Feel Good and Live Long*

Books are available at *www.Amazon.com*

www.ingramcontent.com/pod-product-compliance
Lightning Source LLC
Chambersburg PA
CBHW060205290526
45789CB00003B/1174